# BODYWORKS
## ODES TO OUR ANATOMY

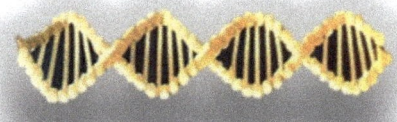

## MARTHA R. HINMAN, PT, DPT, EdD

© COPYRIGHT 2024 BY MARTHA R. HINMAN

ISBN: 978-1-9-965498-39-2

All rights reserved. No part of this book may be reproduced or transmitted in any form or by any means, electronic or mechanical, including photocopying, recording, or by any information storage and retrieval system, without permission in writing from the copyright owner.

The views expressed in this work are solely those of the author and do not necessarily reflect the views of the publisher, and the publisher disclaims any responsibility for them.

**To order additional copies of this book, contact:**

Simply Best Reads LLC
39-67 58th Street, 1st floor
Woodside, NY 11377, USA
Phone: (+1 888-203-7688)
simplybestreads.com

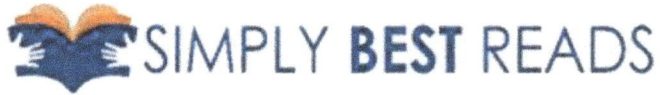

# TABLE OF CONTENTS:

| | |
|---|---|
| PREFACE | IV |
| DEDICATION | V |
| Ode to DNA: The body's blueprint | 1 |
| Ode to the UTERUS: The body's incubator | 2 |
| Ode to the UMBILICAL CORD: The body's first lifeline | 4 |
| Ode to the LIPS: The body's door | 5 |
| Ode to the BONES: The body's scaffold | 6 |
| Ode to the SPINE: The body's erector set | 8 |
| Ode to the NECK: The body's rudder | 10 |
| Ode to the FOOT: The body's foundation | 11 |
| Ode to the HAND: The body's manipulator | 12 |
| Ode to the PATELLA: The body's pulley system | 14 |
| Ode to the BRAIN: The body's generator | 16 |
| Ode to the THALAMUS: The body's relay station | 17 |
| Ode to NEURONS: The body's wiring | 18 |
| Ode to the EYE: The body's camera | 19 |
| Ode to SKELETAL MUSCLES: The body's movers | 20 |
| Ode to the DIAPHRAGM: The body's bellows | 22 |
| Ode to ALVEOLI: The body's diffuser | 23 |
| Ode to the LABYRINTH: The body's gyroscope | 24 |
| Ode to the NOSE: The body's air filter | 26 |
| Ode to SKIN: The body's armor | 28 |

Ode to HAIR: The body's cap _____ 30

Ode to the TEETH: The body's blender _____ 32

Ode to the TONGUE: The body's connoisseur_____ 34

Ode to the INTESTINES: The body's food processor _____ 35

Ode to the LIVER: The body's detox center _____ 36

Ode to the APPENDIX: The body's spare part _____ 38

Ode to the KIDNEYS and BLADDER: The body's plumbing _____ 39

Ode to the HEART: The body's pump _____ 40

Ode to RED BLOOD CELLS: The body's delivery service _____ 42

Ode to our LIFESPAN: The body's clock _____ 44

# PREFACE

What do you get when you cross an anatomy text with a poetry book?

The resulting *BodyWorks* is a collection of odes to God's greatest creation, the human body. It was written for anyone who has an interest in how our body is designed and how each part works. Each poem relates a specific body part to some mechanical tool that helps illustrate its physiological function.

As you read through these verses, you may even formulate some of your own analogies about how your body functions. Nevertheless, the difference between man and machine is an obvious one – the first is a divine creation while the second is a worldly invention.

Fortunately, we are not robots composed of sheet metal, pipes, gears, and wires. Rather, we are complex beings made from the fruits of a Holy Spirit. I hope you will enjoy reading these lyrical odes as much as I enjoyed writing them.

# DEDICATION

Nearly 25 centuries ago, a Chinese philosopher named Mencius reportedly stated that *"Friends are the siblings God never gave us."*

One of my dearest friends is someone who fits that description well. Following her long career as a nurse, transplant coordinator, and hospital administrator, she was recruited to serve as the Executive Dean at Long Island University in New York.

Soon thereafter, I was hired to develop the Doctor of Physical Therapy program at LIU. We formed an instant bond as she was, and continues to be, my strongest supporter and encourager in that endeavor.

She is truly a kindred spirit with whom I can freely share my faith and fascinations, as well as my fears and frustrations. Thus, I lovingly dedicate this literary work to my friend, ***Winnie Mack***, who has always had my back!

~ Martha R. Hinman

# ODE TO DNA:
## THE BODY'S BLUEPRINT

A double-helix structure is my hallmark shape.

And the information I carry helps determine your fate.

Half comes from your father and half from your mother.

That's why not one of us is just like the other.

Will you be a girl or boy, with eyes blue or green?

Will you be short and stout, or tall and lean?

Will your hair be red or blonde or black?

Or maybe hair will be something you lack!

Will you live a long life or will it be cut short?

By some family condition you're unable to thwart?

No one really knows which child gets which trait,

Because I keep it locked in a code that is tough to break!

# ODE TO THE UTERUS:
## THE BODY'S INCUBATOR

What is that wandering around this protected womb?
Could it be an egg looking for a place to bloom?
Look out! Here comes a bunch of invasive sperm,
And they're trying hard to penetrate its ectoderm!

Alas! One of them just got in,
Which means a new life is about to begin.
But how long will this tiny human occupy my space?
Will it need a few weeks or just a few days?

Oh no! Nine months is a long time to house a guest.
I'm not sure I can stretch enough without getting stressed.
It's growing bigger every day and starting to move around,
And other people are watching it with ultrasound.

Now it's beginning to kick which is not very comfortable!
But I won't fight back because I know it's still vulnerable.
However, soon this occupant will be fully grown,
So, maybe I should help it find a new home.

I'll just move things along with some pushing and nudging;
Someone better let those people know this kid is coming!
Think I'll push a little harder now to help deliver this package;
I have to guide it out carefully, so I don't cause any damage.

I feel a sudden rush of energy as my hormone levels surge,
Followed by shouts of joy when this child starts to emerge!
My job is finished now, and I can finally rest —
At least, until another egg lands in
my nest.

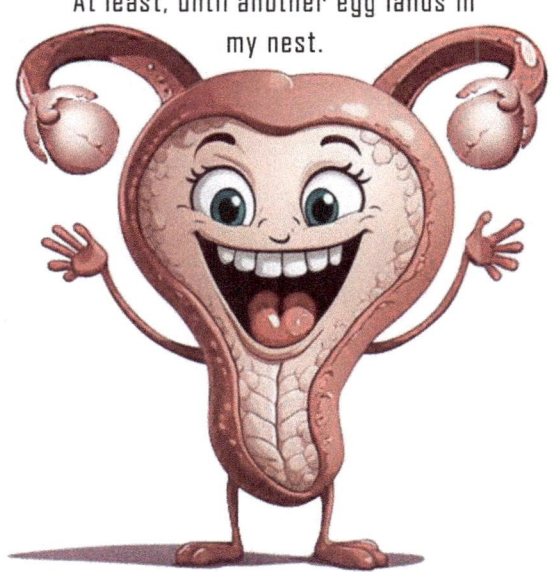

# ODE TO THE UMBILICAL CORD:
## THE BODY'S FIRST LIFELINE

Each time a mother conceives a new child,

A bond is established which allows it to thrive.

Nutrients are delivered from mother to baby

Through a coiled cord which looks a bit snaky.

The two-way channel that exists in this cord,

Ensures that baby's needs are never ignored.

Vital oxygen is received through mom's blood,

Which also removes any of the baby's own crud.

Once the baby leaves its mother's womb,

It is free from the confines of its small cocoon.

It no longer needs the cord's vital protection;

So, with a clamp and scissors, we sever the connection.

But the cord leaves behind a small belly scar,

That might poke in or out, but never too far.

Perhaps it exists to always remind us,

Of a mother's love that continues to bind us.

# ODE TO THE LIPS:
# THE BODY'S DOOR

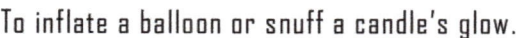

When we two come together,
we work as a pair
To form a smile or a kiss to share.
We can be squeezed more tightly when we need to blow,
To inflate a balloon or snuff a candle's glow.

If you're really unhappy, you can stick the lower one out,
Like children do when they want to pout.
You should also know we have an abundance of nerves,
So, if you're punched in the mouth, it can really hurt!

The muscles that surround us help formulate your words
And control facial expressions that convey your concerns.
At times when you might want to feel more romancy
You can give us more color to make us look fancy!

But if you decide to pierce us with a stud or a ring,
Beware of the problems caused by that sort of bling.
Maybe you should just show off our God-given glamour,
And allow us to function in our own natural manner.

# ODE TO THE BONES:
## THE BODY'S SCAFFOLD

You might say we are the body's greatest rock stars,
Because we hold you together like a bunch of rebar.
And we pose for millions of photos each day
Using x-ray machines that film in shades of gray.

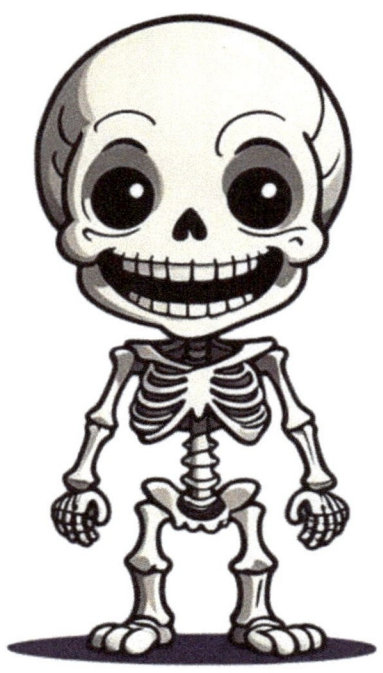

Like puzzle pieces, we come in many shapes and sizes;
When fully assembled, a whole skeleton arises!
Ounce for ounce, we're stronger than steel,
But if we were just as solid, you'd weigh a great deal.

Although our lattice-like structure really lightens our load,
Without the proper nutrients, we can easily erode.
Then we might collapse and cause you great pain
Unless you do something to reduce our strain.

As an adult, you have two hundred and six of us;
And the jobs we perform are rather robust.
When joined end-to-end, we move legs and arms;
And we surround vital organs to protect them from harm.

Our largest pieces are somewhat hollow inside;
In this innermost space is where our marrow resides.
It works round the clock, creating billions of blood cells;
And provides a safe haven for stem cells to dwell.

The smallest of our kind is found deep in your ear;
It controls the vibration from the loud sounds you hear.
Another small cousin floats down under your chin,
Holding onto muscles that help you speak and sing.

Regardless of size, we all have special roles to play,
To keep your body functioning in a healthy way.
Please give us plenty of calcium and Vitamin D,
So we can be the "rock stars" you need us to be!

# ODE TO THE SPINE:
## THE BODY'S ERECTOR SET

My thirty-three blocks support your large skull,
And they connect to your pelvis and legs below.
Without my flexibility, you'd be a walking stick —
You couldn't stretch or bend, and certainly
not twist!

My vertebrae have unique shapes that interlock,
And the disks found between them help absorb any shock.
I'm connected by strong ligaments to ensure my stability,
And my long and short muscles provide lots of mobility.

The space between bones protects a long nerve chain
Which transmits messages from your toes to your brain.
Some attach to the ribs which enclose your chest organs,
And protects them from any unnecessary distortions.

But, alas, my complex structure can easily collapse
When disks dry out and bones start to crack.
Then those nerves get squashed and cry out in pain
For someone to give them relief again!

Some try to stretch me, manipulate me, or apply traction,
While others poke me with needles or inject medication.
As a last resort, a surgeon's hand may be needed
But even surgery has not always succeeded.

So, you must do your best to keep me on course –
Don't jump from high places and land with great force.
Don't lift heavy weights or twist when you flex,
Don't sit too long, and lie down when you rest.

Drink plenty of water to hydrate my disks,
And eat the right food to reduce fracture risks.
Exercise the muscles in your stomach and back,
That should keep me strong, aligned, and intact!

# ODE TO THE NECK:
## THE BODY'S RUDDER

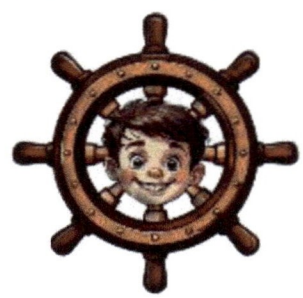

I think it's time I received greater recognition
For my contribution to your sense of direction.
Most people claim that the head directs your path,
While its eyes scan for objects that might cause a crash.

But the eyes can only see what lies straight ahead,
Unless I expand your view, making it more widespread.
It is my flexibility that turns your head to the left or right
And lets you look down at the ground or up at the light.

Without me, your focus would have a definite limit,
Because I'm the one that allows your head to pivot.
My seven vertebrae work together to make me so mobile,
And their combined range-of-motion is really quite notable.

Perhaps that is why the phrase "sticking your neck out"
Is used to describe those who carry great clout.
Because I'm the one who really leads the way,
And keeps you from ever wandering astray!

# ODE TO THE FOOT:
## THE BODY'S FOUNDATION

As body parts go, I don't occupy much space,

But I can propel the rest of you from place to place.

My twenty-six bones give me great flexibility,

And they're connected by ligaments that add some stability.

My heel is very tough because it hits the ground first;

The more you weigh, the more force it must disperse.

But I have a long arch that helps absorb this shock,

And puts a spring in your step each time you walk.

My five toes can provide that extra push you might need,

When you want to run or jump with greater speed.

The muscles that move me are both long and short;

Some move my joints, while others provide support.

Together, we help you maintain your stance,

When you kick a ball, or try to tap dance.

But our greatest distinction among the body's whole

Is that we're the only part that has a real "sole."

# ODE TO THE HAND:
## THE BODY'S MANIPULATOR

What purpose do I have for this bundle of tendons and nerves?

I may be a small part, but I have many functions to serve!

Some say I'm manipulative, while others praise my sensitivity.

My palm lines can predict your fortune, but with some uncertainty.

I can hold onto things tightly or let them go –

I can wave good-bye or say hello!

I can make unfriendly gestures or tell you things are okay;

And I can check you for fever if your health goes astray.

I can hold a pencil when you're learning to write

And you can use my digits to tie shoe laces tight.

If math is a challenge, you can count on my fingers

However, I'm not much help when it comes to large numbers!

I can type a text message on your computer or phone,

Or give you a massage if you're stressed to the bone!

If you ever get angry, my fist can strike a hard blow,

But I'd rather caress gently, with love to show.

My index finger can point the way for your trip;
Or it can silence the noise when raised to your lip.
My thumb is quite handy when you must hitch a ride,
And it can pacify a baby that is starting to cry.

My fourth finger serves a very special purpose
When it accepts a ring during a marriage service.
Although there's not much left for my little pinkie to do
You'll need it if you want to play a fiddle or flute.

Sometimes you need two of us to work as a pair,
Like when we're folded together to lift up a prayer,
Or make signs that allow a deaf person to hear,
Or clap them together when there's reason to cheer.

But of all my talents, there's one I value most,
Because it creates a bond that keeps us all close.
The motion is quite simple and easy to understand –
You just reach out and grasp another person's hand!

# ODE TO THE PATELLA:
## THE BODY'S PULLEY SYSTEM

I sometimes feel so all alone,

Just sitting on top of this large thigh bone.

I've been called a knee cap due to the shape of my surface,

But this term doesn't explain much about my real purpose.

Technically, I'm known as a sesamoid bone,

Which makes me sound like some magical stone!

But I don't perform any tricks, you see,

I just glide up and down on top of your knee.

With my unusual shape, I can't form my own joint,

So, when it comes to movement, I will surely disappoint!

I only attach to one muscle which limits my ability;

Nevertheless, I can influence its strength and agility.

You see, as the knee extends, your quadriceps lose power,
Which makes it hard to hold you as erect as a tower.
But my connection to this muscle enhances its leverage,
And that is what gives it a mechanical advantage.

Thus, I may be small, but I have a big job to do;
And yet, these benefits have their downside too
Because the pressure created when this muscle contracts,
Eventually wears me down, causing my cartilage to crack.

This leads to arthritis which creates some serious pain
When you try to climb stairs and come down again.
Eventually you may need surgery to get some relief;
With a plastic button and metal groove, you can end my grief!

# ODE TO THE BRAIN:
# THE BODY'S GENERATOR

Functionally, I'm what makes you feel cerebral,
And structurally, I'm grander than any cathedral.
Though I look like a convolution of gray and white matter
My billions of nerve cells create a power generator.

I may be 60% fat, but I'm still rather dense,
And my storage capacity is truly immense.
I will shape your personality as you develop and grow,
While you learn new things and make memories to stow.

I process your vision, your hearing, and taste;
And I enable you to sense your position in space.
I control your movement, your appetite and sleep,
And I'm in charge of emotions that make you laugh or weep.

I will focus your attention when a question is asked,
Or allow you to divide it when you must multi-task.
My untapped potential seems to have no limit,
As I harbor your dreams and mold your spirit.

And although your thick skull offers me some protection,
A stroke or head trauma can disrupt my perception.
Fortunately, I'm capable of forging new connections,
Which may help me restore some of your intellection.

# ODE TO THE THALAMUS:
## THE BODY'S RELAY STATION

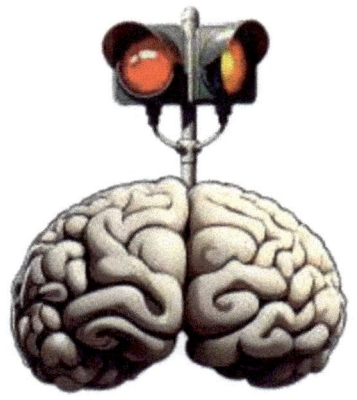

I am best known as the body's relay station,
Because I am constantly transmitting crucial information.
I may be small, but my task is large;
When it comes to communication, I'm the one in charge!

I transmit sensations from your limbs to your brain
And send motor signals down to your muscles again.
I get to decide what's important and what's trivial,
So, you don't pay attention to things immaterial.

I help regulate emotions and memories and learning,
And even the sex you may sometimes be yearning!
But, if I'm disabled by some disease you befell,
You won't be able to think or move very well.

Your hands may tremble and you'll just want to sleep,
And it may be difficult to make sense of your speech.
Because when the brain's traffic signal goes on the blink,
Soon your whole body will be out of sync!

# ODE TO NEURONS: THE BODY'S WIRING

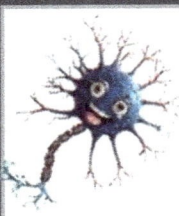 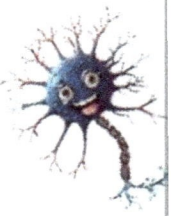

We're the cells that send messages to and from your brain.
We can sense a light touch or deep pressure or pain.
We also send signals that keep your heart beating
And allow you to taste the foods you are eating.

We can excite your muscles and make them contract;
You can see this clearly when your tendons are tapped!
We work in a series much like the wires in your home
With a spark between us to keep the current flowing.

Our electric signals travel quickly along
A very thin fiber we call an axon.
Some are insulated with a myelin sheath,
Which greatly increases their conduction speed.

But if our axonal wires get tangled or frayed,
The signals we carry won't be fully conveyed.
Then your muscles may weaken and your feet become numb,
And you can't think clearly which makes you feel dumb.

Although many conditions can cause our destruction,
Sometimes new connections can restore your function.
This "neuroplasticity" is truly a gift from God,
That should be viewed with a great deal of awe!

# ODE TO THE EYE:
## THE BODY'S CAMERA

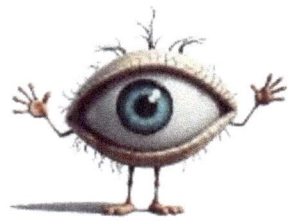

Aye! Aye! I am the eye! I will make your world come alive!
My lens absorbs the light that gives you sight,
And my pupillary hole is like the window to your soul.
My surrounding iris comes in colorful hues,
Such as browns and greens and baby blues.

Aye! Aye! I am the eye! Beyond my lens, the retina lies.
Its rods and cones send signals to the brain,
To interpret and store the image they retain.
The brain takes the visual cues it receives,
And interprets the meaning of whatever it sees.

Is it light or dark? Is it familiar or not?
Is it a thing of great beauty? Or does it look rather gloomy?
Is it a friend or foe? Or a stranger unknown?
Could it be soft and furry? Or is it simply too blurry?
If the brain can't make sense of what is seen,
Then perhaps it wasn't real, but merely a dream.

Aye! Aye! I am the eye! When you're sad, I make you cry.
I can close my lids tight when you sleep at night,
And my blink is quicker than a candle's flicker.
But if ever I'm damaged, and your vision is gone,
You may still view your world through the eyes of a dog.

# ODE TO SKELETAL MUSCLES:
## THE BODY'S MOVERS

Some of us are smooth while others pump the heart;
But most of us have fibers that slide together and apart.
The spark from a nerve will make us twitch,
Like someone who just flipped on a switch.

We attach to your bones and function like levers;
Because moving your joints is our primary endeavor!
We allow you to walk and run and leap;
We let you grasp an object or extend your reach.

There's really no limit to the ways we contract,
Just watch any athlete or acrobat!
We can move quickly with power or slowly with precision;
We can transport you through space or just hold your position.

When we carry a load, it just makes us stronger;
And when you stretch us out, we'll get a bit longer.
Most of the time, we prefer working in synergy,
So, we can perform our jobs more efficiently.

In addition to giving your joints their mobility,
We also ensure your postural stability.
Our long and short muscles support your spine,
To ensure that it stays properly aligned.

Many of us are given other special functions,
Like the ones that control your facial expressions.
Rib muscles assist when you need to breathe deeply,
And pelvic muscles help keep your bladder from leaking.

Our largest muscle provides a cushion for your bottom,
While the smallest one protects your ears from loud volume.
Some of us attach via several long tendons;
Which reduces the bulk in your toes and fingers.

Although our contractions remain under voluntary control,
You're not always aware of our actions or role.
Perhaps your brain just has better things to do
Than to keep track of our each and every move!

# ODE TO THE DIAPHRAGM:
## THE BODY'S BELLOWS

I am the dome-shaped muscle between your thorax and abdomen;
Designed to help you breathe, without thought or intention.
My lower attachment connects through a central tendon
That creates a vacuum with its downward descension.

This motion draws air down into your lungs
Which is how the respiratory process is begun.
The lungs extract oxygen for the blood to carry out,
To energize your whole body before its return route.

Then I can relax, and your lungs can deflate,
Expelling the carbon dioxide they accumulate.
I repeat this cycle about 20,000 times a day,
Although I can work faster if you're running away.

Some folks compare my action to mechanical bellows,
Although I sometimes need help from other muscular fellows.
But whether you are actively moving or calmly asleep;
I'll continue working with the rhythm I keep.

# ODE TO ALVEOLI: THE BODY'S DIFFUSER

Some say we resemble a small cluster of grapes
But we have nothing to do with eating or taste.
We're like tiny balloons that fill up when you breathe,
And extract the oxygen that your whole body needs.

Because our cell walls are extremely thin,
We can transfer that oxygen to our next of kin.
Our capillary relatives on the other side
Take up that oxygen and give it a ride.

The blood delivers $O_2$ throughout the body,
And collects the waste like a porta-potty.
When that blood returns with the $CO_2$ it bears,
It is returned again to the atmosphere.

And so, the cycle continues without conscious effort,
As you breathe in and out at least 12 times a minute.
But if an infection or scarring won't let us expand,
Then we can no longer meet your oxygen demand.

So, avoid contaminants and by all means, DON'T SMOKE!
Because that is the quickest way to make us all choke.
Clean air is a blessing that we constantly seek –
Because pollution and allergens just make us weak.

# ODE TO THE LABYRINTH:
# THE BODY'S GYROSCOPE

Deep inside each of our ears
Are three fluid-filled canals shaped like spheres
Together this web of interconnected hoops
Forms a structure that acts like a gyroscope.

Each canal attaches to a special nerve
That senses in which direction we swerve.
The nerve then signals our head's position in space,
To keep us upright when we move from place to place.

Small hairs are found in each canal's base
That hold tiny stones which act as small weights.
When fluid moves past them, these little hairs bend,
And trigger a message for the nerve to send.

But if a sudden move shakes those ear rocks loose,
You will find that your balance is greatly reduced!
You begin to feel dizzy, like your head took a swim;
And you can't walk straight because the room starts to spin.

Then nausea ensues as your stomach gets upset,
And your eyes may bounce like a marionette.
Technically, this condition is known as "vertigo,"
And, if left untreated, it can cause you great woe!

Fortunately, there's a rather simple technique
That can relocate these stones and provide some relief.
The maneuver is fast and highly effective;
And it requires no drugs to be corrective.

But beware! These symptoms can still recur,
If you get up too quickly when you begin to stir.
Avoid sudden motions that cause those stones to detach,
And please don't engage in a boxing match!

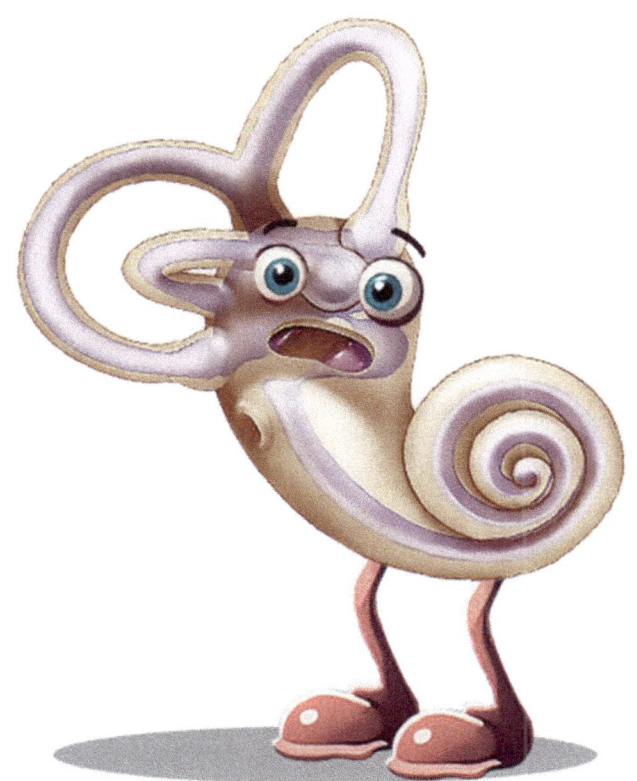

# ODE TO THE NOSE:
## THE BODY'S AIR FILTER

All animals have a structure that protrudes from their face,

Which allows them to smell the aroma of their space.

A squirrel's nose can distinguish its kin from a stranger,

And bunnies will twitch theirs when they sense danger.

A dog's nose has a unique print like the one on your fingers,

And they can pick up any scent as long as it lingers.

But the animal that has the greatest sense of smell

Is the elephant whose long trunk is full of smell cells!

Although the human nose detects far fewer scents,

Its primary function is one of defense.

With all the pollutants that are found in our air,

We're lucky to have a filter in our nares.

Occasionally we inhale germs or some kind of virus,

That generates a strong sneeze to clear out our sinus.

And when certain allergens cause our nose irritation

We may need to rid them with nasal irrigation.

But sometimes our noses will still get congested
With all the pollen and dust that we may have ingested.
Then its mucous will likely begin to f ow
Until we clear it out with a very hard blow!

If you're unfortunate enough to wind up in a brawl,
A punch to your nose makes it hard to breathe at all!
And because it's so vascular, your nose easily bleeds,
Unless you stuff it with cotton to help stop the stampede.

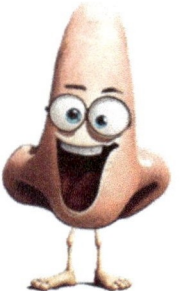

Besides its function for smelling and breathing,
Some noses can actually make a face more appealing.
Of course, if you have one that's too large or very crooked,
You might need some help from a good plastic surgeon!

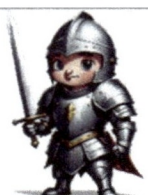

# ODE TO SKIN:
# THE BODY'S ARMOR

Which organ is the largest – did you guess the liver or brain?
It is actually your skin which covers a lot more terrain!
Depending on your size, it occupies about 20 square feet,
And accounts for 15% of your total body weight.

Although you shed skin cells on a daily basis,
It constantly makes new ones to maintain homeostasis.
And it acts as an armor against environmental invaders
That constantly try to penetrate its numerous layers.

Not only does its barrier enhance our immunity,
But our skin's imprints give us our unique identity.
And its color helps characterize each person's race
Which tends to vary from place to place.

It contains cells that protect us from the sun's hostile rays
And allows us to sweat on those hot, humid days.
If we get cut, burned, or scratched, it is amazing to see
How quickly skin repairs itself and gets rid of debris!

Aside from its critical role of protection,
Its flexibility allows joints to move in any direction.
And skin provides nutrients to grow nails and hair;
Without them, our fingers and head would be bare!

But probably the skin's function that we don't think about much
Is its ability to provide us with a keen sense of touch.
Skin receptors send the brain precise information
Such as deep pressure, light touch, or a painful sensation.

Without our skin, this body would certainly not last;
Every part underneath it would deteriorate fast.
So, don't subject it to needless wear and tear;
Our skin will fare well if we give it great care!

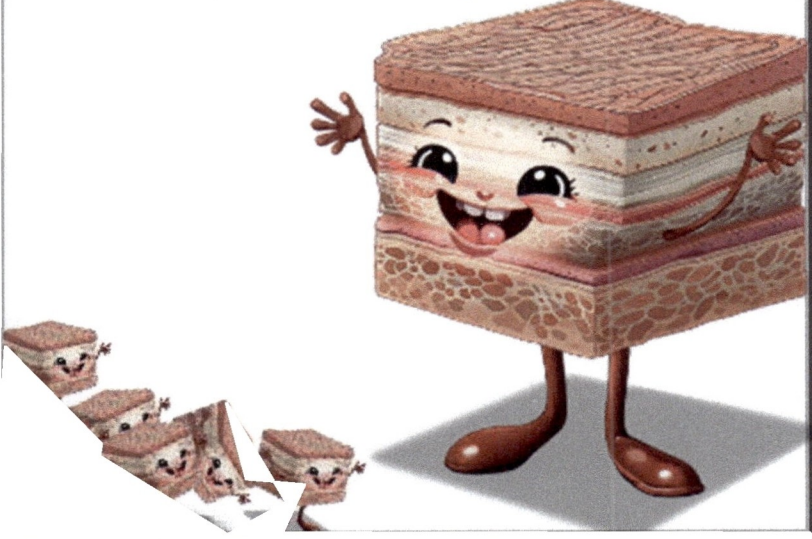

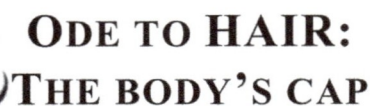

# ODE TO HAIR: THE BODY'S CAP

We can be thick or thin, short or long,
Straight or curly, brown or blonde.
Our variability makes your physique more unique.
We can even give you a nice widow's peak.

Although you may lose over 100 of us each day,
We are replaced very quickly and without much delay.
If you never trim us, we'll be long and flowing;
But, eventually we would all just stop growing.

Our strength is sometimes compared to steel,
Though our flexibility doesn't provide much building appeal.
But when braided together, we create a strong, flexible rope,
Like the one Rapunzel's prince was able to grope!

What does our color say about you?
There are many myths surrounding our hue!
Some say blondes are the most flirty and fun;
Others think redheads are the more passionate ones.

Black hair is most common and marks a serious thinker,
While brunettes tend to be loyal hard-workers.
But if your strands are colored pink, purple, or green,
You probably don't like anything that's too routine!

Eventually our color fades as most people age;
Some claim its appearance is the mark of a sage.
Others fear it's a reminder of our mortality;
Maybe that's why the Bible calls us "a crown of glory"!

# ODE TO THE TEETH:
## THE BODY'S BLENDER

Our enameled surface is the hardest part of your body.
But without proper care, we can get holes and look shoddy.
We aren't visible in newborns and may disappear when you're old,
But in between you will see us whenever your lips unfold.

We come in various shapes, from molars to incisors;
As you mature, we add some to make you wiser!
Together, our goal is to assist you when eating;
Our sharp, jagged surface can give food a real beating!

If ever you're threatened, we can also offer protection,
By chomping down on whoever acts with aggression.
However, a punch in the mouth could cause us to loosen,
And, in some cases, that might disrupt our occlusion.

Quite often our surface will lose its white color;
Then we no longer sparkle and begin to look duller.
Other times we grow crooked or develop too much clearance;
Then we need a dental expert to restore our appearance.

Simply put, we are the first thing most people will notice
When you meet someone new and make their acquaintance.
So, our job requires more than just biting and chewing;
We must make a good impression when a relationship is brewing!

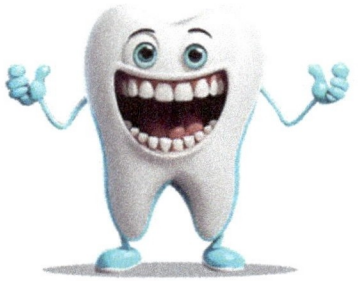

But eventually, as old age takes advantage of you,
We might begin to fall out, leaving behind just a few.
Fortunately, we aren't really that hard to replace;
With dentures or transplants, we put a new smile on your face!

# ODE TO THE TONGUE:
## THE BODY'S CONNOISSEUR

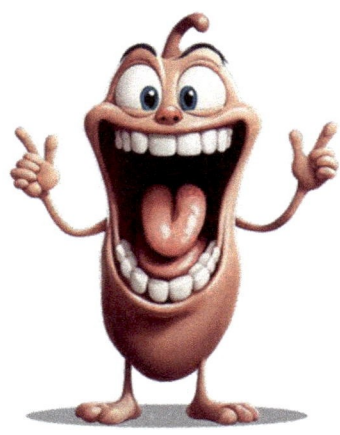

To what do we owe this unique oral muscle?
It can't lift a weight or give us the power to hustle!
But it secretes saliva which helps soften our food,
And we can express dissatisfaction when we make it protrude.

It helps form words so we speak with distinction,
And its taste buds produce many flavorful sensations!
It tells us whether food is salty, sour, or sweet,
Or warns us if something's too bitter to eat.

It's an expert at licking a lollipop,
Or enjoying a cone with ice cream on top!
But the most sensual role this muscle can play
Is the pleasure it provides when we kiss the French way!

# ODE TO THE INTESTINES:
## THE BODY'S FOOD PROCESSOR

When fully outstretched, we may be 30 feet long,
But curled up in your abdomen is where we belong.
Our smaller part helps break down your food,
And absorb the nutrients once they've been unglued.

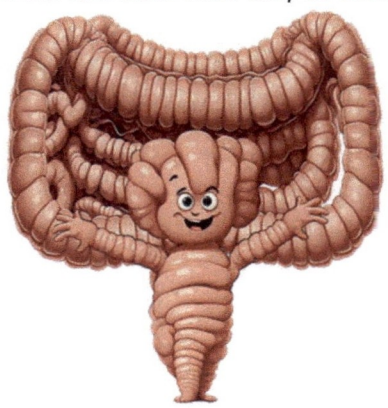

The remaining mass is passed on through
To our larger half which knows what to do.
With the help of bacteria, it extracts important vitamins,
Like the K and B types, including one called biotin.

With the leftover fiber, we form poop that must pass
On through our colon, along with some gas.
If you stop to consider what we might think,
You'll probably agree that our job really stinks.

As body parts go, we have little beauty and grace,
So why do doctors enjoy viewing our inner space?
All that poking and prodding feels so intrusive –
Too bad we can't make ourselves a bit more elusive!

# ODE TO THE LIVER:
## THE BODY'S DETOX CENTER

My numerous jobs make me quite the multi-tasker!

If I didn't work so hard, your body would be a disaster.

I remove nutrients from your blood to generate energy,

And store extra vitamins in my vast organ treasury.

I produce glucose, proteins, and vital hormones,

That regulate blood pressure along with the growth of bones.

I can generate enough heat to keep your body warm,

And my bacteria-fighting cells are always ready to swarm!

My protection also includes the removal of toxins

That cling to various drugs and alcoholic concoctions.

But the most unique talent that I alone possess

Is my ability to regenerate when I'm overly stressed.

Nevertheless, sometimes I am scarred beyond repair;

Then, the only help left may come from a prayer.

Although a transplant can provide a surgical option,

Not many of us are really up for adoption!

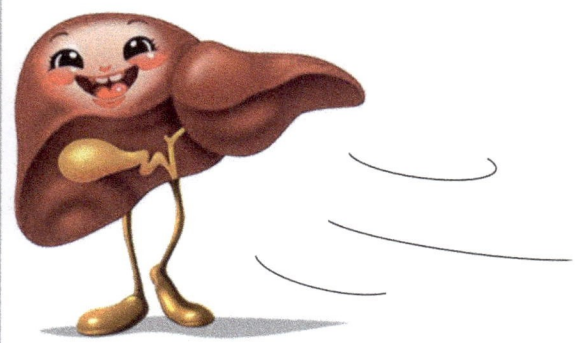

A better way to ensure my consistent good health
Is to consume foods that keep me spry as an elf.
I'm quite fond of fibrous veggies, berries, and oily fish;
Fresh coffee and tea also make my list.

So, be a liver lover and treat me with respect,
And I will deliver everything you expect.
I will energize, mobilize, and always protect,
By removing those toxins that make your body a wreck!

# ODE TO THE APPENDIX: THE BODY'S SPARE PART

Some say I'm useless
and just want me removed,

But I must have had some purpose
when this body was approved!

Although I'm part of your gut,
I don't help your digestion,

But I do store good bacteria
which needs my protection.

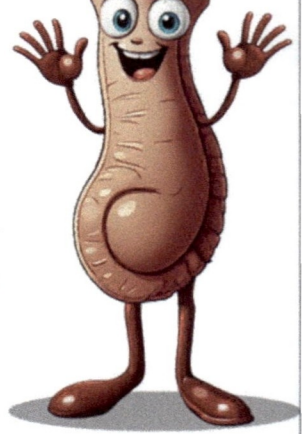

When attacked by illness,
I can release these do-gooders,

And let them rid your intestines
of nasty intruders.

Just beware that if I become
too stuffed and stressed,

I might swell or burst and cause great distress.

Then I suppose you will clearly know

That it is really time for me to go!

# ODE TO THE KIDNEYS AND BLADDER:
## THE BODY'S PLUMBING

Every time you consume some liquid refreshment,
It is used to hydrate every organ and segment.
Eventually, there will be some fluid to spare,
But it can't be stored just anywhere!

It flows through your blood and
into the kidney
That filters out toxins and
clears away the debris.
Leftover fluid drains into the
bladder's sac,
Where it is held until you're ready
to unpack.

Its walls are lined by a special smooth muscle
That easily stretches because it's so supple.
But when that muscle is stretched to its limit,
It will begin to contract, and that will make you fidget!

Then you'd better pay attention and seek some relief
Or that plumbing of yours will soon spring a leak!
It's much like the stress we keep bottled up inside;
But some activity and prayer should help it subside!

# ODE TO THE HEART: THE BODY'S PUMP

I don't understand how I gained such popularity
And became known as the body's greatest celebrity.
I am symbolized by a distinct color and shape
And I'm the subject of marriage and spiritual debate.

I have my own holiday in the month of February
When cards are shared along with tasty confectionary.
The world seems to think that I generate love
But that emotion actually comes from above.

Some claim I can be cold but that's simply not true –
I'm always warm since I'm inside of you.
And I don't really break the way some think I do,
Because I'm tough enough to withstand a blow or two.

You see, I'm just a thick muscle that acts as a pump
To deliver life-sustaining blood with every thump.
I work 24/7 without rest or delay,
Beating over 100,000 times each day.

If I occasionally stop and cause you some pain,
An electric jumpstart should restore me again.
And if the valves inside me begin to leak,
You can replace them with new ones that aren't so weak.

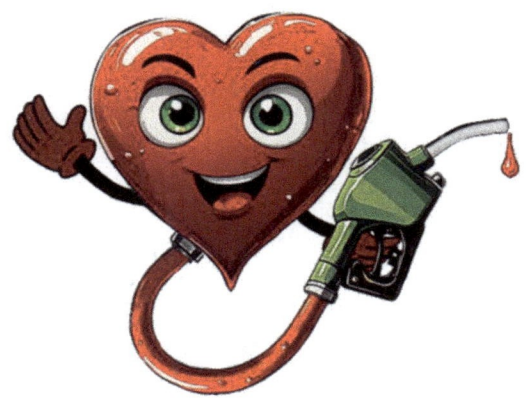

So, the next time you speak about "matters of the heart"
Don't forget what really sets me apart!
Because you won't last long without my steadfast support,
And whether you're in love or not, that would make your life short.

# ODE TO RED BLOOD CELLS:
## THE BODY'S DELIVERY SERVICE

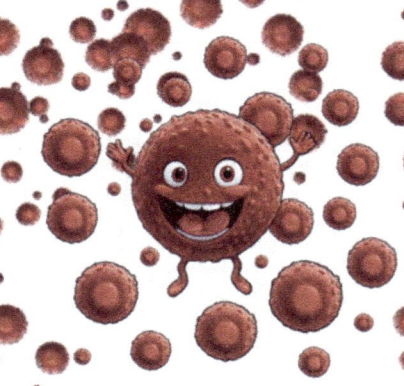

We are red and round and with oxygen abound;
To energize every tissue and organ around.
We deliver our cargo with a speed that astounds,
Traveling 60,000 miles daily is truly profound!

No other delivery service can boast such a record,
And none can compete with our extraordinary effort!
Though we only live for 120 days,
We never stop – even for holidays!

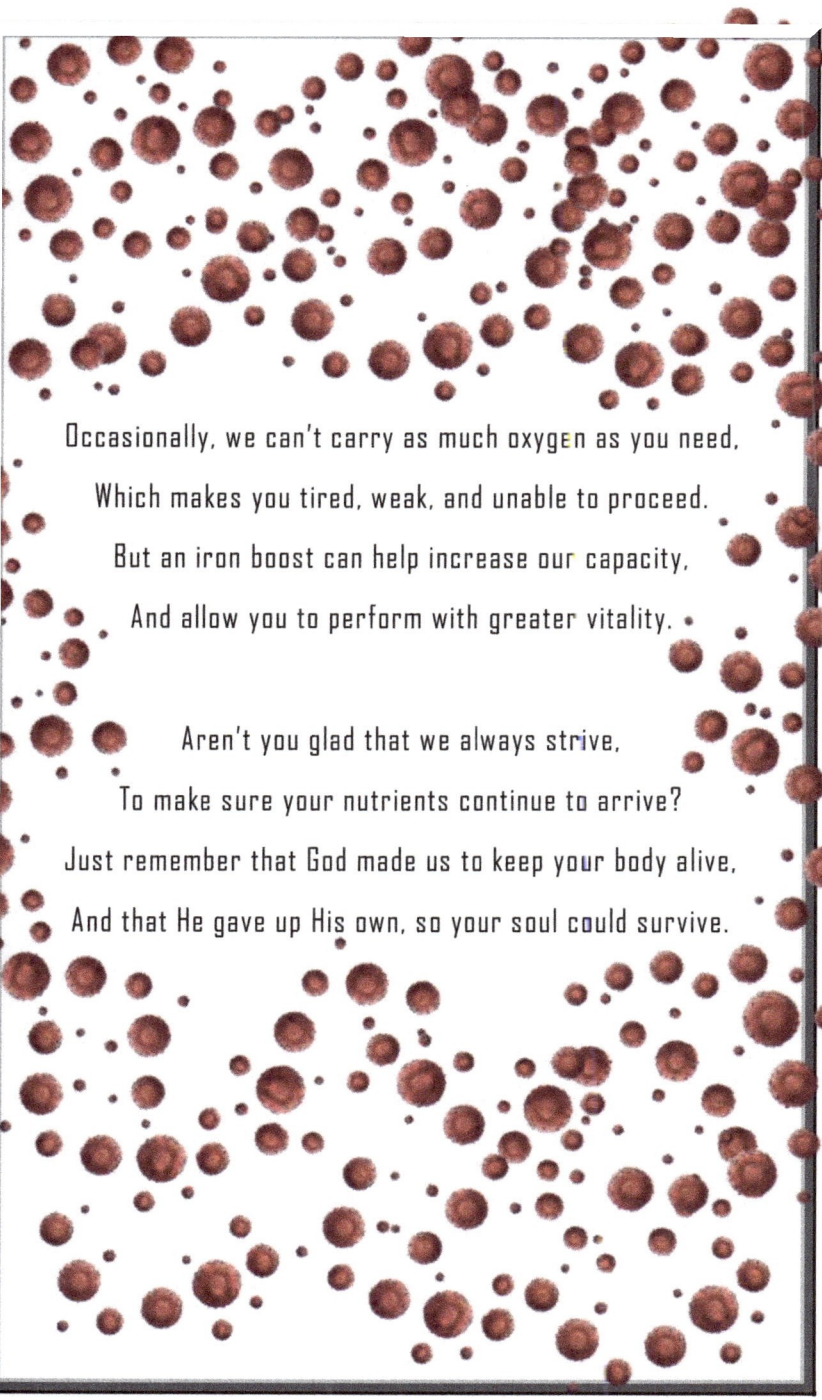

Occasionally, we can't carry as much oxygen as you need,
Which makes you tired, weak, and unable to proceed.
But an iron boost can help increase our capacity,
And allow you to perform with greater vitality.

Aren't you glad that we always strive,
To make sure your nutrients continue to arrive?
Just remember that God made us to keep your body alive,
And that He gave up His own, so your soul could survive.

# ODE TO OUR LIFESPAN:
# THE BODY'S CLOCK

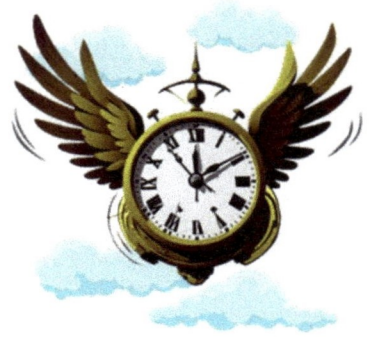

Our lives begin when two cells unite,
And create a new being that is too small for sight.
As cells rapidly divide, a head and spine emerge
With arms and legs that begin to diverge.

When that infant is ready to greet the world,
It leaves the womb and becomes uncurled.
During the next several years, it will grow in size;
And though it learns fast, it is still not too wise.

When it reaches maturity, its strength will peak,
But within a few years, those muscles grow weak.
Its bones become brittle and its hair turns gray,
And its balance develops a little more sway.

Its skin becomes thin while its eye lens gets thicker,
Its reflexes slow down, and its joints become stiffer.
The heart still pumps, but it's not as efficient,
And its hearing can be rather insufficient.

So, what's left for this older being to enjoy?
Is there anything these years cannot destroy?
Rest assured – old age still has its perks;
It can nap when it wants to and eat lots of desserts!

There's time to reflect on all the memories it made –
The love that was shared and the ideas it conveyed.
Until it's time to leave this worldly space,
And find a new home in a more heavenly place.

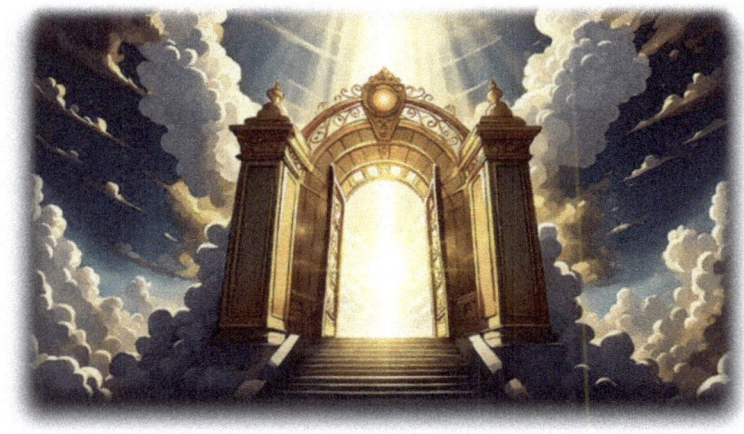

www.ingramcontent.com/pod-product-compliance
Lightning Source LLC
LaVergne TN
LVHW050137080526
838202LV00061B/6512